Mindful Minds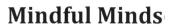

Daily Devotions Power of the Super

By: CWEN STARR SHELDON

TABLE OF CONTENTS

If you're like most people, life hasn't always been smooth sailing for you - in fact, you've probably endured setback after setback, emotionally draining fiascoes and being dumped on unfairly. So now it's time to put all that pressure and heat to good use and adopt the Success Mindset by embracing your diamond mind!

Think about it for a minute... One of the most precious gems in the world today is a diamond, right? Yet those glorious, sparkling, sought-after diamonds began their journey as simple, cheap coal. That coal was transformed by pressure and heat until it was molded into diamonds - it was the constant, long-term pressure and incredible heat that turned a cheap commodity into an item of great value.

The same can be said of your own mind, if you so choose. All of that stress and pressure you've dealt with has given you a wealth of experience in dealing with whatever life throws at you. Being under fire at work, in social settings and/or at home has taught you tact, diplomacy, humility and the benefits of holding your tongue. And when you put those two together, you gain a lot of new wisdom - just think about how much wiser you are now than you were ten or twenty years ago.

To go back to our example, not all coal becomes diamonds. In fact, it's precisely because there are so few diamonds that they've become so valuable. And it's the same thing for people in the general public - most are average and run-of-the-mill, but a select few in every generation are really spectacular. What makes them stand out isn't IQ, breeding or wealth - it's mindset.

Embracing Your 'Diamond Mind' Mindset

Fortunately, every person has the ultimate control over their mindset. But you have to take active control of your own mindset or you'll default to a frame of mind dictated by outside sources like television, online media, politicians and worse. If you're currently living in the 'Life Sucks' camp, it's a safe bet you're accepting someone else's version of reality instead of embracing your own diamond mind!

People with real self-confidence and a lot of energy tackle every challenge with gusto and succeed a lot more often than they fail. You've probably looked on such people with some mix of envy and dislike - never realizing that changing your mindset could make you one of those over-achievers too.

Where does their self-confidence come from? It starts from realizing all they been through has taught them a lot - including how to handle future challenges. And for all the world has thrown at them, they're still standing...

Well, isn't that true of you too? The more you've been through to this point, the deeper the well of experience you have to draw on and the better you know how to handle anything life throws at you in the future. Trust in that wisdom & your diamond mind to overcome your challenges on a going-forward basis.

Each new challenge becomes another victory, adding to your self-confidence and your motivation - and that ever-increasing motivation is the root of more and more energy as you move forward in life! And as you move forward along this cycle you'll reach critical mass, with energy and self-confidence at self-sustaining velocity.

You, too, can stand out in any crowd just by remembering - and using - all you've survived and all you've learned from your experiences to date. Use your diamond mind mindset to really thrive and tackle each day with the confidence that you'll be triumphant once again!

MINDSET ANALYSIS

Life is effort-return phenomenon. People make efforts to actualize returns. There is nothing more frustrating than putting in lots of effort and getting no desired results. The secret to the wasted efforts lies dominantly in a person. A survey indicated that 75% of businesses are failed in their initial phase, first 3 to 5 years, and the major reason of business failures, about 90%, are executives. They are not genuinely prepared for the task in hand. In addition, an established business may also decline or can produce less than optimal results due to negative mindset or stagnant behavior of executives.

Human behavior is predominantly the outcome of his/her mindset. Mindset affects the actions of a person and outcomes of efforts, having a negative mindset or even a neutral mindset can distort the actions and undermine the efforts. How it works? Answer is simple, whenever a person possesses a negative mindset, he radiates negativity. Negativity means pessimism, despair, and disinterest. It compels people to avoid/dislike/misinterpret him. Moreover, when a person is negative, he tends to see only hurdles and magnify them. And when someone sees only hurdles or magnifies hurdles wrongly, he tends to feel stress. When a person is feeling lots of stress, he can't be sensible or creative. Therefore, a negative mindset undermines rationality creativity, dynamism, and productivity. In contrast, a positive mindset allows someone to deal with inevitable challenges with rationality, creativity, dynamism, and resourcefulness.

The complete positive or negative mindset is a special phenomenon. In real life, we come across with partial positive or negative mindset. A person may be positive at some situations or negative at some other situations. However, its effectiveness is normally misunderstood and misused. We make an effort to comprehend its nature, importance and significance for its better usage.

Definition

Suppose there is a glass. It is half full or empty with water. If we take a small survey and ask about the water situation in the glass, there would be two true answers:

- First, glass is half full with water,
- Second, glass is half empty with no water.

It is said that the group of persons mentioning it half full are optimist or have positive mindset; on the other hand, the other group is pessimist or have negative mindset. It is not right conclusion. Both statements are true or scientific. The positive or negative mindset is indicated when a person delivers a statement about or respond with some predictable exactness / exaggeration. A mindset refers to a framework of intentions, perceptions, and emotions held by a person so established that predetermines a person's response to and interpretation of situations /persons.

Negativity Traps

We take a few real life situations to fully grasp the concept and the characteristics that make up a negative or positive mindset:

- A person faces a surprised situation/person and feels envy but responds with jealousy, it is indication of negative mindset. The other examples of jealous mindset are - happy response on someone's miseries, sad feelings on someone's success, & defamation of opponent. (Jealousy)

- A person faces a disliked situation/person and responds proudly without any scientific basis, it is indication of negative mindset. The other examples of proud mindset are -

perfectionist approach, slavery of habits, and dictatorial stance during decision making. (Proud)

- A person faces a new situation/person and takes it with doubts without any scientific basis; it is indication of negative mindset. The other examples of doubtful mindset are - doubt about personal strengths, expect failures, and doubt on ground realities. (Doubt)

- A person faces an unexpected situation/person and considers it a threat without any scientific basis; it is indication of negative mindset. The other examples of fearful mindset are - fear of future, fear of criticism, and fear of failure. (Fearful)

- A person faces a novel situation/person and loose mental stability and responds with volatile attitude; it is indication of negative mindset. The other examples of volatile mindset are - lethargic response, impatient behavior, whimsical decision making. (Volatility)

- A person faces an unfavorable situation/person and loose self control and responds with anger; it is indication of negative mindset. The other examples of unjust mindset are - under or over estimations of abilities, excessive criticism on mistakes, and mild response on blunders. (Injustice)

- A person faces a new situation/person and feels frustration and respond with grief sentiments; it is indication of negative mindset. The other examples of grief mindset are - overwhelmingly critical behavior, pessimism, and disbelief on real success. (Grief)

These examples indicated seven major negativity traps or vicious circles of mental framework that make up a negative mindset. The solution to avoid the vicious traps is to develop a mental framework with positive intentions, positive perceptions, and positive emotions.

Mind Anatomy

Naturally human mind has two sides - left and right. The left side is logical, analytical, and critical. On the other hand, the right side is intuitive, creative and synthetic. The left side is problem seeker while the right side is problem solver. Both sides have their own importance and significance. In addition, we have two levels of mind - conscious and subconscious. The subconscious mind is filled with energy and power to accomplish multiple insurmountable tasks but is led by our conscious mind. Conscious mind makes selection from continuous stream of thoughts (negative & positive) and develop a working pattern or belief system for subconscious mind. It is a continuous process of selection and execution remain active in everyone's life.

Unfortunately, negative thoughts have a tendency to flit into our conscious mind, involve left side of mind turning down the right side of the mind, do their damage and then flit back to continuous stream of thoughts; the significance of process is generally unnoticed. In addition, we hardly perceive them as negative thoughts; we do not challenge them properly so that they may reside in our mind and can distort our mental framework, now and then. Fortunately, the same process is with positive thoughts. They blink in our conscious mind, involve both sides of mind, without letting down any side of mind, do their constructive work and flew back to thought stream. It is hardly to notice them and to harness for permanent constructive activity. By noticing, captivating, maintaining, and protecting a positive thought, we can make them a permanent part of our mental framework for everlasting fruitful results.

Mindset is combination of intentions, perceptions and emotions. It has three powers for execution, i.e., will power, intellect power, and emotional power. These powers are essential ingredients of our mind. Equilibrium is necessary for the stability of mind pyramid; however, e uilibrium may be wise or positive and unwise or negative.

MINDSET DEVELOPMENT

We have learned the mind anatomy with negativity traps that make our life miserable and unhappy. We can move now towards positive mindset. To avoid negativity traps, self suggestion is considered the best technique for mindset development. The words and phrases of self-suggestion should be real, constructive, energetic and dynamic. By continuous repetition we can make a positive image of self. A person can make his own list; however, we mention a few quotes:

- Anything fruitful for humanity will must realize sooner or later,
- Any right effort with right intent and methods will must produce good results,
- There is no real/permanent threat only opportunities,
- Any misery has blessing in disguise,
- Success is not pursued, it is attracted,
- Gratitude brings benefits,
- Patience is best and fruitful strategy in difficulties, and
- Courtesy costs nothing but buys everything.

Any positive suggestion is reacted by negative suggestion. A war is started in mind about these self suggestions with negative suggestions. The process remains active until a belief is not finalized. A belief may be negative or false and positive or true. A negative belief about something/someone, e.g., life is aimless, no real relationship is possible, the hells are always the others, success is impossible, miseries are permanent, benefits are short-lived, and difficulties are long lasting. A negative belief produces or breeds new negative beliefs and a negative belief system is developed. A negative belief system plays havoc with an individual or system or society. A scientific / factual approach is strictly needed to avoid a negative belief system. There are two tested weapons for negative suggestions - Knowledge and Wisdom. Knowledge is a weapon used at conceptual level to counter negative suggestions/beliefs, while, the wisdom is applied at practical level. A suggestion based on knowledge and wisdom would be free from negativity traps. It is noteworthy that a rational person can make errors but not systematic errors. We learn from past errors / other's errors and adjust our beliefs and actions accordingly.

Example

We take an example from socio-economic life to establish and internalize the whole concept. It is three steps road map towards positive mindset - Thought Awareness, Rational Limitation, and Self Suggestions.

Step - I (Thought Awareness)

Suppose you are going for some presentation / negotiation. There are some typical negative thoughts you might experience about presentation / negotiation:

- Fear about the quality of performance, technical problems that may come up, and harsh criticism;
- Worry about the reaction of peers, general audience, and stakeholders;
- Doubt on real strengths / potential opportunities,
- Visualizing the negative consequences of a poor performance;
- Self-criticism over less than perfect preparation, rehearsal and practice,
- Frustration or Anger on certain real inadequacies or deficiencies.

These negative thoughts / negativity traps can damage confidence, harm performance, paralyze mental skills, and radiates negativity.

Step - II (Rational Limitations)

In rational limitation process you challenge the negative thoughts and counter them with rationality. Looking at some of the examples, the following challenges could be made to these common negative thoughts:

- Quality of performance: Have you gathered the information you need and prepared it properly for the event? Have you conducted a reasonable number of rehearsals, real or mental? If so, you've done as much as you can to give a good performance.

- Technical Problems and issues outside your control: The key to develop a rational limitation for successful presentation / negotiation on technical problems is to realize that you cannot control all relevant factors in your presentation / negotiation that may create a distraction. While you can control your own behavior or your organizational skills, you cannot control traffic jams, airline delays, power shutdown, computer network outrage, and communication problems due to damaged e⊡uipment. However, it is important to consider the possible risks and necessary steps to mitigate their effects.

- Fear about harsh criticism / Worry about other people's reaction: If you perform the best you can, then you have given a good performance, fair people are likely to respond well. If people are not fair, then the best thing is to ignore them and rise above any unfair comments.

- Problems during practice: If some of your practices were less than perfect, then remind yourself that the purpose of practice is to identify problems so that they will not be repeated during the performance. Similarly, ask yourself whether it is reasonable to expect perfect performance. All that is important is effective/great performance not perfect.

Step - III (Self Suggestions)

By now, you would be more positive. The final step for effective positive mindset is to prepare self-suggestions to counter any remaining negativity. Continuing with the same example, some positive affirmations could be:

- Quality of performance: "I have prepared well and have rehearsed thoroughly. I am ready to give an excellent performance."

- Problems of distraction and issues outside your control: "I have thought everything that might reasonably happen and have planned how I can handle all likely contingencies. I am well equipped to react flexibly to any surprised situation."

- Worry about other people's reaction: "Fair people will react reasonably to a well-prepared performance. I will rise above any unfair criticism in a mature and professional way."

WHY POSITIVE THINKING WORKS

Positive thinking does create positive outcomes. But not everyone believes that. Some people think positive outcomes are only dictated based on how much effort you put into something. And, while effort counts, how great of an outcome can you have if you think miserably along the journey to that outcome? Some people think positive thinking is a "trendy thing" and that the truth is, "whatever is meant to be will be." And while destiny, fate, etc. can be something to believe in, you must realize that your mind and the energy you give off impacts that destiny. And then, you just have cynical people that always find the bad in situations or play devil's advocate way too much. Well, that is their prerogative, don't feed into it and stay away from them.

If you want more positive outcomes in your life, you do have to think positive. Positive thinking steers your course into a positive outcome. Here are ways positive thinking leads you toward a positive outcome:

Positive Thinking makes you See More Resources.

Happy and positive people see what they do have, and that goes for their resources, too. Those who think limitedly, are cynical or fail to see the positive in situations often miss resources that are right around them. They often close their mind to their community and those around them who want to help. You may often hear them use the statement "I always do everything myself." This is a very powerful black and white comment. This type of thinking shuts down a lot of amazingness right around them. Instead, the positive minded person looks at the resources they do have even if they are limited. They will work harder to find resources in the community that could support them. Resources will help you gain momentum, stay your course, and help you hurdle barriers. All things that will lead to a positive outcome.

Positive Thinking Builds Confidence.

When you think positively you think positive about what is around you. You see the good in life and in people. You trust in yourself and your resources. This process builds confidence. As you see the strength and goodness of your world and yourself, you are more apt to take healthy risks. Instead of letting fear stop you from huge dreams and goals, you are able to believe in yourself and take leaps toward goals. You know that if you hit a barrier, you can hurdle it or those around you will help you hurdle it, and that builds confidence. Confidence is what you need to take risks and risks often lead to positive outcomes, like success.

Positive Thinking Keeps You Open-Minded.

Positive people have open minds. They listen to others, not just give their two cents. This gives insight into what people desire, what questions they should ask and alternate points of view. They try to see life through different perspectives. By opening your mind, you see more answers, opportunities and ways to live your life fully. More opportunities, more insights and more fulfillment create more positive outcomes.

CREATING A MINDSET FOR SUCCESS

Success is a choice and choosing to be successful - in family life, in business, in relationships, in health - is a matter of deciding to set goals and attain them. Reaching goals does not have to be an overwhelming prospect, though. Creating a mindset that welcomes success is about taking small steps toward a larger objective.

A Fixed Mindset can Impede Progress

According to Carol S. Dweck, author and professor at Stanford University, success or failure is directly related to one's mindset. She contends that individuals are either fixed-minded or growth-minded. A fixed mindset categorizes personal traits like intelligence and character as unchanging or etched in stone. A growth mindset determines that traits and qualities can be improved with effort. Individuals operating with a fixed mindset often find it difficult to advance in their careers, are ineffective in leadership positions, and are generally more pessimistic about life. They are unable to admit when they are wrong and do not adapt to change well. Those with a fixed mindset cannot gauge their own abilities accurately, feel that their current intelligence level (and the intelligence of others) is permanent, are frequently judgmental, and are unable to read other's ability to change.

This is not to suggest that those with a fixed mindset are any less interested in advancing or succeeding than their growth-minded peers. "The irony of a fixed mindset," says Dweck, "is you want to be so successful so badly that it stands in the way of going where you want to go."

Overcoming a Fixed Mindset

Often, a fixed mindset is the result of years of personal experience or emotional trauma that has caused psychological pain or doubt in one's worth. The seeds are planted in childhood or adolescence and may be very difficult to overcome. As perceived disappointments mount, the negative or defeatist mindset compounds until an individual believes this perception to be reality. Achieving success and true fulfillment requires amending a fixed mindset. The process must begin with a period of intense self-evaluation.

Question deeply entrenched personal beliefs. Examine self-image and identify ways in which the subconscious mind limits success or growth. Pay attention to the inner voice that prevents progress or complicates goal-setting. For instance, an individual wishes to lose weight. If he is of a fixed mindset, his inner voice will constantly flood his subconscious with reasons why he is wasting his time - the holidays are coming and the weight will just come back, there is too much going on at work, it will require too much effort, it will never work, etc. Conquering this kind of self defeat is crucial to obtaining success.

The next phase in the process is to focus on a goal. Whether it is to get a better job, be happier in one's marriage, be a better parent, or buy a bigger house, the goal should be something significant and meaningful. Once a large goal has been established, create a path to that goal by plotting several smaller goals along the way. These mini goals represent tangible, attainable steps that will eventually lead to the main objective. Breaking substantial goals into stages reduces the weight of achieving what is truly desired and puts success closer at hand by situating many little victories along the way. This generates a sense of encouragement that keeps an individual focused upon the process; the main goal is reached organically, without much of the trepidation and disappointment of past attempts.

The man who wants to lose weight may set a smaller goal of taking a 10 minute walk after dinner every evening for an entire week. At the end of the week, he might set a new goal of a 20 minute walk every day for the next week. Each week is another victory and by the end of a month he's lost ten pounds. In taking these specific, manageable steps toward his main goal he is quieting the negative inner voice that was overwhelmed by the vague idea of losing weight.

Priming for Success

Once those negative inner voices have been quieted, it is still necessary to open oneself to the possibility of success. This is especially true for those who have long believed themselves unworthy or ill-equipped for achievement or fulfillment.

Many individuals believe it is possible to train the mind in a new reality through positive affirmation and visualization. By repeating goals aloud or imagining a desired outcome, one can prepare the mind to be more receptive to change and to welcome it when it occurs. In this way, success gradually becomes an expected outcome, not something unusual or unlikely. Failure is transformed from an embarrassing circumstance or a defeating experience to an opportunity for learning and growth.

There are three central components to preparing the mind for success. These are gratitude, faith, and purpose.

- Having a gracious attitude toward individuals and situations allows one to find peace. One is able to let go of the past and learn from mistakes, grateful for the chance to have obtained an important lesson or to have had a particular experience.

- Nurturing a strong sense of purpose allows individuals to have full control over their futures and to set the terms for their own destiny. This creates a sense of power and ownership that is not easily defeated by the self, by others, by circumstance, or by setback.

- Faith is also important, and not necessarily the spiritual or religious type. Having faith in oneself and in one's abilities is critical in building a link between past experience, present circumstance, and future goals. Trusting that change is possible is the driving force behind achieving success, no matter how dire the current state of affairs may seem.

Putting it into Practice

Altering one's mindset is a constant, ongoing process. It is important to work diligently to maintain progress and to strive for further development. Encourage gratitude by acknowledging the present situation for what it is, and admit that no matter how bad it seems it could have been worse. Be thankful for the way events have unfolded and learn relevant lessons that will cultivate future success.

Fortify a sense of purpose by frequently setting goals, no matter how insignificant. Contemplate the things that are important and be brutally honest about what is truly desired. For some, it helps to write down these goals or discuss them with others. Keeping one's wishes and desires at the forefront of consciousness ensures that one's sense of purpose is never in danger of wavering.

Strengthen faith by practicing self care. This can be achieved through daily meditation, spiritual pursuits, physical activity, reading and writing, artistic endeavors like painting or sculpting, and any other way in which the self is nurtured and one's self-confidence is boosted.

No matter how deeply ensconced one's fixed mindset or negative self-image may be, there is always opportunity to silence the inner critic and open the mind to success.

CHANGE YOUR MINDSET BY FOCUSING ON OPTIMISM

Stop Focusing on the Negative

If you want to be successful the first key in doing so is to change your mindset. You have to be SELF AWARE. Stop focusing on the negatives and start focusing on just the positives. When you get mad you stay mad because you continue to think those negative thoughts. You're essentially adding more fuel to the fire for yourself making you more upset. People dwell and dwell on all the bad things that occur, but don't ever stop to recognize any of the good that happens. People push themselves harder and harder, but never stop to pat themselves on the back.

To say "think positively" may sound like a cliché statement, but most cliché statements tend to be true. Once you catch a bad thought circulating in your mind then that is the best time to catch it, change your perspective and change your mindset.

Whatever it is that you tell yourself which keeps you trapped in your comfort zone is what you need to change. In order to change something you have to alter it meaning do something completely opposite of what your mind tells you. Here's a common example, you see people having fun and dancing at a wedding. You want to dance too but a thought tells you that you'd look ridiculous and you restrict yourself from doing so. Instead of letting that thought control you, tell yourself you only get one life and you want to live it like it's your last. If you BELIEVE and feel the raw reality and rationality behind that thought then your mood and perspective alters. Slowly you regain confidence and off you go.

To change your mindset identify your own thoughts you tell yourself and really examine them. Don't over think things but internalize whether or not this thought is driven from a rational or self-limiting perspective. If it's a self-limiting perspective ignore it and focus on the RATIONAL. If you continue to focus on your negative thoughts you'll doubt yourself later down the road which will hinder your road to success. The only way to break a habit is through repetition and learning to change your mindset is no different. Anything that hinders clear thinking in your mind will surely hinder your success.

Understand your Destination and Set yourself a Path

Everyone has something that motivates them to push harder. Some have their children, others have their family, and some just have themselves. If you want to establish success you have to clearly lay out the foundations and steps towards reaching that overall destination. If you want to change your mindset the one thing that tends to motivate others to push themselves harder is happiness. People have many definitions and ways of achieving happiness and I like to think that everyone's goals should consist of a much larger purpose other than money even if that includes pursuing that "feeling of happiness". If you want to help others than you should set consistent financial goals to help move you closer and closer towards your humanitarian journey. Life has a much larger purpose and materialism is not and never will be the answer. Find something that drives something within you and slowly you'll start to change your mindset, this is a true tool of success.

Once you've established a foundation that motivates and pushes you forward you have to clearly lay out your goals. How are you going to get there? You have to lay out every single detail to develop a road map towards your destination. Your goals have to be measurable and reasonable. Don't over push yourself. When your creating your goals just note that you should be doing something PRODUCTIVE at all times. Develop daily, weekly, and monthly goals to accomplish on a consistent basis. Set long term goals to help push you and set short term goals to keep you on your feet. Never stop until you reach those goals. In order to change your mindset you have to create a foundation and establishing your path is just the beginning.

Actually sticking with those goals is going to be the hard part. Staying consistent is going to be the only way you'll develop a habit and discipline is the habit you'll need in order to change your mindset.

Focus on the Moment

Focusing on the moment is just a natural part of life. The beauty of everything happening all at once still gets me wondering. In order to be successful you have to have a clear mind. In order to do that you have to NOT BE THINKING. Actually process what's going on NOW. When your minds not scattering all over the place you feel more in touch with reality and with yourself. When you're constantly thinking, your mood starts to get affected from certain thoughts or reactions. This hinders your progress of changing negative thinking since negativity is usually triggered by a thought. Focus on your goals and the smaller goals you've set up to help get you there and anything else direct your attention towards the moment. Focusing on the moment is how true inspiration strikes and it's vital in order to change your mindset.

Journal

The only way to track your progress is through journaling. By journaling you record and recollect on what your conscious and subconscious mind thinks. If you have heard the saying your only using 10% of your brain than imagine what you can uncover by journaling. When you journal you can internalize your own deficiencies and negative thoughts a lot more clearly. When you're conscious, your mind is circulating different things and usually people are not so in touch with themselves that they can stay aware of every single thought that crosses their mind. The whole goal of journaling is to see how your mind reacts to certain events and identifying how you can alter that pattern so in the future you can create a different event, situation, thought, or opportunity and change your mindset.

Journaling is extremely calming. After you let everything out you feel cleansed and a lot more at peace because journaling is a form of self-therapy. Journal every day and practice consistency because overall this will help you with discipline and in identifying negative patterns.

SIMPLE STEPS TO SHIFT YOUR MINDSET FOR SUCCESS INSIDE AND OUT

As spiritual beings living in a physical body we have all the resources needed to achieve and do anything we want in business and life. These (resources) tools are your thoughts and beliefs. The truth is you can use your thoughts and beliefs to create anything you want in life.

The challenge is a lot of what we think and say is ?uite limited or negative and do not create a good experience for us. So, to shift your mindset for success inside and out, the key is to change the beliefs we hold in our minds, the negative or limiting thoughts that come to our mind even though most of us know that they are not true.

Using the tool I'm presenting here, what is called: "Affirmation" opens the door for your new way of thinking and seeing things that support your growth in business and life. This tool is just a starting point so you can begin to change the thoughts you have in your subconscious mind.

The reality is what you are really doing is saying to your subconscious mind that "I AM in charge, I'm AWARE that I can change; I'm taking the control of my life." When I'm talking about doing "affirmations," I'm suggesting to choose specific words that can help you eliminate something you do not want to create, and instead choose what you DO want to create - something you REALLY want in your life.

From my own personal experience, I've realized that every thought I have and every word I say is an affirmation. You and I are using affirmations whether we know it or not, and most importantly we are creating everything in our lives using these affirmations.

My recommendation here is for you to start paying attention to your thoughts so you can start to eliminate the thoughts that do not support you in your journey during your time here on Earth. For example, every time you think "I do not want poverty," you are attracting more poverty to your life. If you have a thought that ""life is not supporting you," what you are really saying - putting out in the universe - is that you are not living the way you should live. I suggest you to change the way you talk to yourself. If you have negative or limiting thoughts in your mind, it does not mean that you are not a good person or that you cannot have what you desire, what you need to do is to change the way you talk to yourself.

Probably you talk the way your parents talk and your parents learned to talk the same way your grandparents talk. Most likely your parents taught you how to talk and you also learned a lot of things from the environment you grew up. Nobody is wrong but it is time for you to consciously choose your thoughts that really support and please you. If I can do it, and many people have done it, so can you.

Some people say that affirmations do not work which it is an affirmation itself. What they really mean is that they do not know how to use them correctly. They may say "I'm getting healthier" and the voice inside say "It is stupid and it will not work." Which affirmation do you think will win? The negative one, as it is a long stand part of a habitual way of looking at life.

Affirmation can be compared to seed and soil; if you plant a seed in a poor soil it may or may not grow. The more you choose to think thoughts that make you feel good, and more important that really goes deep emotionally, the faster the affirmation works.

Now, today you have the power to choose the thoughts you are thinking. Your negative or limiting thoughts will not disappear completely in one day, but if you consistently think thoughts that make you feel good, enlightened, you will definitely start making changes in every area of your life.

Here's the thing: we have only one time we are in control of, we have only one time we choose to feel good and this time is NOW. The 'now' is the only time we realistic live in. If we do not live well at this moment, how come will we live happy in the future? We do not have control of the past and the future, the only moment we have control of is the now. If we do not choose to feel good in this moment how can we create future moments that are abundant, successful and fun?

How do you feel right now? Do you feel good or bad? What kind of emotions are you feeling? Would you like to feel better? If so, choose a better thought. What you decide to think is what you will get in life.

Doing affirmations is consciously choosing to think certain thoughts that will create positive results in the future. Affirmative statements are going beyond the reality of the present into the creation of the future by the word you use now. For instance, you may have very little money in the bank, but when you affirm "I am prosperous," you are planting a seed of prosperity into the future. Each time you affirm it, you are nourishing the seed into your mind. After a period of time, your mind will do whatever it has to do to grow that seed. Things grow much 🗆uicker in a fertile rich soil than in a poor soil.

Now you may be asking. How can I use affirmations to start shifting my mindset for success inside and out, and eventually change my life to a more prosperous, joyful and harmonious life? To help you do just that, I'd like to share with you four simple steps that you can apply immediately and get great results today.

Simple Steps to Shift Your Mindset for Success Inside and Out

Be aware of your thoughts.

The first step to shift your mindset for success inside and out, and therefore change your life is to be aware of your thoughts. Awareness is always the first step. When negative or limiting thoughts come to your mind, instead of trying to stop them and waste a lot of energy and effort, ignore them and use an opposite thought.

Shift your negative or limiting thought to an opposite, abundant thought.

After being aware, conscious of your thoughts, the next step is to shift this negative, limiting thought to an opposite, abundant thought. More important, use only thoughts that are aligned with your goals, dreams, passions and purpose, start shifting from limiting thoughts which make you feel anxious, worried and frustrated, to all those unlimited thoughts that make you feel good, abundant and successful inside and out.

It's a great idea if you do not spend any time questioning negative or limiting thoughts. After step 1 you'll be aware of your negative or limiting thoughts, so immediately change the 'thought' with an affirmation that is the opposite of that negative or limiting thought, doing so you'll start attracting things that are aligned with your true unlimited thoughts.

Use present tense, ALWAYS!

Your affirmations MUST be stated in the present. For example, "I have" or "I am." If you say, "I will have," it will stay in the future. The universe takes your words very literally the way you say what you want. So use present tense, ALWAYS!

Repeat the affirmation as often as possible.

You can choose to do your affirmations anytime of the day. However, the best time to do them is before going to bed in the evening so your subconscious mind will work to make your affirmations your reality while you are sleeping.

Here are some good examples of affirmations to help you start creating positive results in business and life right now:

- I live my life with passion and purpose.
- I have an abundance of clients flowing to my business.
- I love and appreciate my body.
- Money flows into my life in an abundant way.
- I allow my body to return to its natural and vibrant health.
- I can do whatever I set my mind.

Every positive thought brings good into your life, every negative thought pushes good away. So why not choose a prosperous, joyful, beautiful, lovely thought that will make you feel good? The choice is YOURS.

HOW TO HAVE THE MINDSET FOR SUCCESS

Learning how to have the mindset for success is crucial when you want a successful and blissful life. If you are like me, you might have many goals you want to achieve. Whatever these goals are, the key is to have a growth mindset rather than a fixed one. But what is the difference and how you get it?

How can you set and have the mindset for success? Do you want to reach your goals more rapidly? In how many years did you plan to achieve your goals?

Many people, as well as I, preach hard work, focus, persistence and more but these are by-products of something else. It is something much more powerful than we can all develop. This extraordinary thing is critical to success, and it is your mindset.

Without the right mindset, you might find yourself sidetracked by your everyday routine. You can also often be distracted by the latest and most fabulous idea you are just having, which rarely pushes you to follow one path until successful.

You may think that you have all the time in the world to achieve your goals. But you have to realize that if you set your mindset for success, you can apply it to other domains as well. In this way, you will reach your goals much faster and find yourself with the capacity to possibly form new and bigger goals.

The Trap of the Mindset

It is always better to fail many times before succeeding as it will help you avoid many of the psychological traps. One of the key traps is to believe that you are smarter than other people, or that you do not have to work hard because you have talent, or that you have nothing to learn.

To have the right mindset to be successful in life, you do not need to have extraordinary intelligence or be gifted with talents.

"The moment you believe that success is determined by an ingrained level of ability, you will brittle in the face of adversity." - Josh W., International Chess champion.

So, as soon as you think success is determined by talent, you become weak when you have to face obstacles.

The Difference between a Fixed and Growth Mindset

So as soon as people see intelligence or abilities as fixed, they believe that many things are impossible for them to achieve because they put limits on themselves and their skills. And that is what is called a fixed mindset.

But other persons see abilities as qualities that can be developed which is, in this case, called a growth mindset. The important part is that those two different frames of mind lead to not the same behaviors and results.

When you have a growth mindset, you know you can change your intelligence, and increase your aptitudes and skills over time. But people with a fixed mindset do not think it is possible. So, the difference between the two groups is the perspective on intellect and brainpower.

The Possibility of a Different Mindset

Many studies have shown similar effects for the mindset about any ability such as problem-solving, playing sports, managing people or anything else you would like. The key to success is not merely effort, focus or resilience, but it is the growth mindset that creates them.

Your mindset is critical. When you directly are trying to build determination or persistence, it is not nearly as effective as if as addressing the mind frame that underlies these traits. How many people think of themselves as not creative people, or sociable, or math oriented, or even athletic?

On the other hand, some people may think that they are naturals. But if you want to fulfill your full potential, you need to start thinking differently. You have to realize that you not chained to your current capabilities and that you can modify your mindset.

A Mindset Can Be Changed

You should know that your brain is very malleable and has plasticity. You can change your ability to think and to perform. In fact, many of the accomplished people of our era were thought by experts to have no more future. People like Charles Darwin, Marcel Proust, and many others but they along with all high achievers such as Mozart to Einstein built their abilities.

But the vital thing here is to realize that you can change your ability and picture yourself where you want to be. When you have a growth mindset, you bring your game to new levels. So, how does a growth frame of mind do that?

Well, there are biological manifestations to mindset. Tests show that with people who have a fixed mindset, the brain becomes most active when they receive information about how they perform. Whereas people with a growth mindset, they have their mind being most active when they receive information about what they could do better next time.

The Choice of a Growth Mindset

In other words, people with a fixed frame of mind worry the most about how they are judged while those with a growth mindset focus the most on learning. There are other conse uences about outlook. A fixed mind sees effort as a bad thing, something that only people with low capabilities need while those with a growth approach see effort as what makes them smart and as a way to grow.

And when they hit a setback or failure, people with a fixed mindset tend to conclude that they are incapable, so to protect their ego, they lose interest or withdraw. It is often taken as a lack of motivation, but behind it is a fixed frame of mind.

Whereas, people with a growth frame of mind believe that setbacks are a part of personal development. They find a way around the problem. So it means that you have to challenge yourself. But it also says that you have to praise yourself for being great at something or being smart; so do not also forget to honor others and even children for the same things.

Mindset Affects Everything

Trying hard pushes you to work even harder next time you face a challenge. Do not get into the fixed mindset of thinking that when you win, you are a winner and when you lose, it must make you a loser. The reason being is that your mindset affects your performance.

Remember that you can change your mindset any time you wish. And that is important because many people have a fixed mind frame about something or another. When you teach or have a growth mindset, not only it improves you as an all, but it also narrows down the achievement gap.

Mindset affects all of us. In the workplace, managers and supervisors with a fixed mindset do not accept feedback as much, and they do not mentor people. A wrong or right frame of mind even touches relationships, sports, and health.

Why do schools not teach the growth mindset to children rather than being so critical?

Tips to Have the Mindset for Success

- Get a growth mindset.
- Develop Success Habits.
- Recognize that a growth mindset is beneficial.
- Know that your brain changes when you work hard to improve yourself.
- Make a small step toward each of your goals each day.
- Learn how to develop your abilities as well as teaching others.
- Capture all of the information that could help you.
- Do a deliberate daily practice to develop your abilities through effective effort.
- Listen to audio books or learn a new language on your phone while you are out for a walk rather than music.
- Clip articles and inspiring ideas for a vision board.
- Learn from your failures by asking yourself what you learned from the experience.
- Know your strengths and weaknesses.
- Develop core skills that will help you reach and achieve your goals.
- After experiencing a setback, do not dwell on it. Instead, make an evaluation, and move on to the next thing.

DISCOVERING THE POWER TO SUCCEED IN POSITIVE THINKING

Positive thinking or attitude conditions the mind, with thoughts, words and images that will bring about the actions required for the desired results. Positive mental attitude desires and expects good and favorable outcome (positive results). A positive mind anticipates happiness, joy, health and a successful outcome of every situation and action. Whatever the mind conceives to achieve, it finds a way to achieve it.

A majority of people do not apply positive thinking in their lives. Not everyone is aware of such a practice or believes in positive thinking. Some consider the subject as just nonsense, and others scoff at people who believe and accept it (e.g. of negative attitude bringing on negative results). For those who accept it, not many know how to use it effectively to get results. Yet, it seems that many are becoming attracted to this subject, as evidenced by the many books, lectures and courses about it. This is a subject that is gaining popularity. Recent good examples that encourage the practice of positive thinking are shown in books like:"The Secret" and "Chicken Soup for the Soul."

It is ❑uite common to hear people say: "Think positive!", to someone who feels down and worried. Most people do not take these words seriously, as they do not know what they really mean, or do not consider them as useful and effective. How many people do you know, who stop to think what the power of positive thinking means? The difficulty in people embracing this is in our tendency to accept negatives easier than to be positive because sometimes to be positive re❑uires a person to fight against his natural tendencies.

According to an author, Mary Lore: "how do we know if a thought is powerful or not? Very simply, by noticing how we feel as we think a thought. When a thought is not working for us, we don't feel good as we are thinking the thought. Our head and neck are tense, our eyebrows are furrowed, our breath is short, our chest and stomachs are tight.

"When we are thinking a powerful thought, we feel good. We feel at peace. We feel a sense of inner power. We feel inspired." This is the power of positive thinking.

The following story illustrates how this power works:

Ashley applied for a new job, but as his self-esteem was low, and he considered himself as a failure and unworthy of success, he was sure that he was not going to get the job. He had a negative attitude towards himself, and believed that the other applicants were better and more qualified than him. Ashley manifested this attitude, due to his negative past experiences with job interviews.

His mind was filled with negative thoughts and fears concerning the job for the whole week before the job interview. He was sure he would be rejected. On the day of the interview he got up late, and to his horror he discovered that the shirt he had planned to wear was dirty, and the other one needed ironing. As it was already too late, he went out wearing a shirt full of wrinkles.

During the interview he was tense, displayed a negative attitude, worried about his shirt, and felt hungry because he did not have enough time to eat breakfast. All this distracted his mind and made it difficult for him to focus on the interview. His overall behavior made a bad impression, and conseＺuently he materialized his fear and did not get the job.

Kently applied for the same job too, but approached the matter in a different way. He was sure that he was going to get the job. During the week preceding the interview he often visualized himself making a good impression and getting the job. In the evening before the interview he prepared the clothes he was going to wear, and went to sleep a little earlier. On day of the interview he woke up earlier than usual, and had ample time to eat breakfast, and then to arrive to the interview before the scheduled time. He got the job because he made a good impression. He had also of course, the proper qualifications for the job, but so had Ashley.

What do we learn from these two stories? Is there any magic employed here? No, it is all natural. When the attitude is positive we entertain pleasant feelings and constructive images, and see in our mind's eye what we really want to happen. This brings brightness to the eyes, more energy and happiness. The whole being broadcasts good will, happiness and success. Even the health is affected in a beneficial way. We walk tall and the voice is more powerful. Our body language shows the way you feel inside.

Whether it's Positive Thinking or Negative Thinking they are both contagious.

All of us affect, in one way or another, the people we meet. This happens instinctively and on a subconscious level, through thoughts and feelings transference, and through body language. People sense our aura and are affected by our thoughts, and vice versa. Is it any wonder that we want to be around positive people and avoid negative ones? People are more disposed to help us if we are positive, and they dislike and avoid anyone broadcasting negativity.

Negative thoughts, words and attitude bring up negative and unhappy moods and actions. When a person's mind is negative, it brings about more unhappiness and negativity. This is the way to failure, frustration and disappointment. Where do negative attitudes come from in the first place?

Negative attitudes come from thinking negative thoughts over and over until they have become a part of your subconscious - they've become habitual, a part of your personality. You may not even realize you have a negative attitude because it's been with you for so long. Once you have a bad attitude, you expect failure and disaster. This expectation turns you into a strong magnet for failure and disaster. Then it becomes a vicious circle. You expect the worst - you get the worst - your negative beliefs are reinforced - you expect the worst - you get the worst. You get the picture?

So, How Do We Shift Our Thoughts And Create A Positive Attitude?

It takes work, but creating anything of value takes work. In order to have a new attitude we have to change our subconscious thinking. How do we do this? By analyzing every thought we have until positive thinking becomes habit. You're merely replacing an old habit with a healthy habit, much like replacing exercise for smoking. You can't just stop being negative - you have to replace those negative thoughts with positive ones.

Some people would say, "But negative situations are a reality. They just show up in every day life." This is absolutely not true. Situations are a reality, yes. They do show upbut it is your ATTITUDE that makes a situation positive or negative. It's time for you to realize that YOU are in control of how you think and feel - no one else on earth has this power unless you give it away. Take control of your attitude, and you take control of your results.

"Your state of mind creates the state of your results."

Some Practical Suggestions.

In order to turn the mind toward the positive, inner work and training are required. Attitude and thoughts do not change overnight.

Get hold of at least a copy of Positive Thinking by Norman Vincent Peale or all his books related to this subject. Read them and learn the important points, think about the benefits and persuade yourself to try it. The power of thoughts is a mighty power that is always shaping our life. This shaping is usually done subconsciously, but it is possible to make the process a conscious one. Even if the idea seems strange give it a try, as you have nothing to lose, but only to gain. Ignore what others might say or think about you, if they discover that you are changing the way you think.

Always visualize only favorable and beneficial situations. Use positive words in your inner dialogues or when talking with others. Smile more as this brings about positiveness. Disregard any feelings of laziness or a desire to quit. If you persevere, you will transform the way your mind thinks and the way you conduct your life.

Once a negative thought enters your mind, you have to be aware of it and endeavor to replace it with a constructive one. The negative thought will try again to enter your mind, and then you have to replace it again with a positive one. It is as if there are two pictures in front of you, and you choose to look at one of them and disregard the other. Persistence will eventually teach your mind to think positively and ignore negative thoughts.

In case you feel any inner resistance when replacing negative thoughts with positive ones, do not give up, but keep looking only at the beneficial, good and happy thoughts in your mind.

It does not matter what your circumstances are at the present moment. Think positively, expect only favorable results and situations, and circumstances will change accordingly. It may take some time for the changes to take place, but eventually they do.

TIPS TO POWER YOUR MINDSET AND GAIN MORE SELF CONFIDENCE

Self confidence plays such an important role in our life on a daily basis. Most of the time we just go on with your day without ever thinking about how confident we feel about ourselves - that is, until we're faced with a huge decision or we need to perform a certain task and expect to do it well.

So creating a solid mindset to feel completely confident anytime and anywhere becomes a very important quality that we can apply to most situations before they ever occur, thus making those challenging moments so much easier to contend with and to help us feel better about them.

For most of us, trying just one method to gain confidence and maintain a confident mindset doesn't always prove to be the best solution, but using a combination of several techni?ues may provide exactly the key outcome to successfully achieve our ultimate goal.

Here are 10 strategies to the solutions that can be used alone, or in a combination to create or change your mindset to gain the self confidence you deserve. (not necessarily in order of importance).

- One of the first and most important concepts to the creation of a strong and sound mindset is to begin with a clear slate. In other words, to erase those obstacles from your past that continue to form negative beliefs which keep you from feeling confident. It's pretty difficult to move forward if you are constantly haunted by negative experiences from your past.

  You can start the healing process by writing down all those past influences that continue to make you feel inade?uate, indecisive, and insecure. I like to refer to this as clearing your mindset closet. Once you've discharged these destructive experiences, you can begin to create new positive associations that will propel you to new horizons.

- Another destructive behavior is to focus on negative situations and outcomes. If you tell yourself that bad things always happen to you, then your subconscious mind will continue to find ways to reinforce that and constantly remind your thought process that "this is just the way it has been and there is nothing you can do about it".

  So this destructive thought pattern becomes the norm and you'll have a very difficult time getting away from this type of behavior (in my book, The 51st State, I refer to this as 'stinkin-thinkin'). Of course, not everything is going to produce a positive result for you, but you can DECIDE that negative outcomes are merely lessons to which you should view as a sign to try a new approach.

  Don't let your mind say to you; "see, I told you only bad things happen" - keep thinking that way and most likely, they will.

- So, with a clear head and a positive attitude, you can begin to create your positive belief programming by some very powerful and influential techniques to disrupt a negative situation that occurs anytime, anywhere.

  Be prepared to change your environment, or enhance the mood, or by documenting the cause so you can avoid a similar outcome in the future. You can put on some loud and fun music, you can go for a walk or run to exert some energy, you can listen to inspiring messages (i.e. my audio session) to help empower mindset and deal with a situation better, or take a hot bath to relax you physically.

Decide for yourself, what works for you to Ɖuickly change the immediate circumstances and you will open new channels to overcome these challenges.

- Create a vision (dream) board that you can look at constantly. This is a great way to form positive beliefs and give you a physical "goal getter" to refer to first thing in the morning, last thing in the evening, and anytime in between.

You can use a bulletin board, white board, electronic graphic on your computer, or a simple cardboard poster that you can attach pictures, quotes, and goals as a constant reminder of what you want, who you want to be, and how you want to feel. Just remember to use this inspiration as often as possible.

Look at it, read it, study it, dream it, and believe in it. You can gain some huge confidence in yourself when you create some visual goals.

- Surround yourself with positive energy. As obvious as this sounds, I'm amazed how many people continue to let destructive influences into their life from others. Join a group of like-minded people that you can relate to and share with and that empower you, or start one.

Stop hanging around those individuals that suck your energy from you and bring you down. Start associating with those you lift you up and energize you and you will probably find yourself with more confidence.

There is so much great opportunity to build confidence when you truly relate to others who recognize your strengths and talents instead of those who want to steal your dreams. Think back on those pivotal moments when someone you met made a huge impact on your life (in a positive way of course) and realize that this can, and probably will happen again.

Set your own boundaries and limits about who you will let become part of your circle of influence and you can feel the incredible power of confidence.

- Getting busy with physical exercise (only with doctor's permission) is probably one the most empowering methods to build self confidence. I have heard from so many people that this is the one thing that really makes them feel incredibly confident physically, mentally, and emotionally.

Sure, you may seek to build muscle, lose a few pounds, look fit, but it's the mental aspect that has a huge impact on building confidence. Just knowing that it takes motivation and perseverance to get out and exercise is very satisfying by itself. Stick with it for awhile, and you should realize some really great physical results from your efforts. It's also a great stress reliever and tension reducer.

There are many ways to get active, from going to the gym, to walking around the block, to working out at home with simple weights or a cardio dvd. You don't have to set huge milestones to shoot for and accomplish at first. Start out with small, achievable goals in the beginning and continue to increase your workout program until you reach your ultimate results. Find something that you can do physically on a regular basis and you can gain the confidence you desire from this terrific form of activity.

- Accomplish something, no matter how insignificant it seems, that gives you some satisfaction that you are moving in the right direction. Confidence comes from results - usually positive results.

  Don't just sit around and wait for things to come your way. Get up and call someone, or open a business account, write a blog post, clean the closet, even plant a garden, something that is necessary to help you move forward.

  There certainly are no guarantees that is will provide instant success for you, but it keeps the motivation factor progressing and hopefully will lead you to the next task to accomplish to reach your goals (you better have some goals).

- Develop some mind-healthy habits of positive reinforcement. Most of us have read motivational quotes to some degree. They can be found all over our busy world, from television commercials, to inspirational wall hangings, to fortune cookie messages, to seminars and programs you can listen to anywhere you go. That's terrific.

  There is such a vast amount of really great messages to keep us inspired all the time. Now, we just have to channel them into our subconscious mind so we create (or change) our belief system. Just reading a great quote or hearing a positive message usually isn't enough to really embed that positive idea firmly in our mind so that we can call on it when we need to.

  Try affirmations, mantras, and meditation, that can have a lasting result and provide a positive memory bank that we can tap into at will. A more consistent approach is usually required to create this part of NLP (neuro-linguistic programming). Put these words of confidence anywhere you spend a lot of time at or on a regular basis.

By reading these powerful messages constantly, you can begin to create your own beliefs that will flush away negative thoughts and replace them with empowering and confident ones.

- Be grateful, thankful, and appreciative of the gifts you already possess. You may be asking; how is this going to give me more confidence? The solution is that we can take a step back and realize who we already are, what we've already accomplished, and what we already have in our lives.

We all have certain gifts that we should be so thankful for. Sometimes it's hard to think about them when we are struggling with life's challenges. This is a great time to make a list of our wonderful traits and characteristics and pin them up on our dream board so that we can refer to them when life becomes difficult.

Confidence in our ability to appreciate the things we have instead of constantly striving for more can have a profound effect on our mindset. That also leads to rethinking what we really want and who we really want to be. Take some time to write down your gifts and be confident with them.

- Never, ever give up. That means never give up on your dreams, your beliefs, or your talents. There is a time when you may be smart to let go of something that is draining you mentally, physically, emotionally, and financially so you can move on to more progressive tasks that will propel you forward in seeking your ultimate success.

You can usually decide when this time is appropriate when it just feels right to part from something that stops you in your tracks or takes too much away from you. It may be a relationship, a j.o.b., a business venture or a destructive circle of influences.

You should be focused on that which gets you closer to success by helping you accomplish your tasks and reach your goals. Sure there will be unexpected challenges along the way, but don't let them bring you down and away from your dreams. You can just expect that challenges will happen, but you can also prepare for some of them by thinking ahead to what is presented in front of you.

Prioritize your tasks, contact those you need help from, and always take some action to get you closer to individual goals.

Try applying as many of these methods to increase your confidence and you may experience a higher power never felt before. Your mindset is so important to your confidence levels, which in turn helps you make decisions, take action, and venture out of your comfort zone, that can lead to the road to realize your ultimate success.

- Focus on making things happen that move you forward and stop wasting time on things that are nonproductive. Confidence crushers are found too easily and in so many aspects of life so weeding through them can prove to turn confidence levels positive by eliminating those things that are destructive.

CONCLUSION

As you know, each of us is different, so it is quite important that you structure your day in a way that works for you. First of all, you should observe your daily routine and be honest with yourself by looking if you do have a productive mindset or if you are just being busy, and correct that.

To be productive means that you are clear minded and focused on what you want to accomplish. It also means that you are using all of your resources to achieve your goals profitably. The next step involves morning habits that would help you get more done through the day.

To continue creating a productive mindset, you have to choose which vital assignment to start doing when you sit down for work. You have to make the right choices so you can kick off your day with dynamic momentum.

Finally, whether you are already committed, wandering on the path of least resistance or basking in the waters of procrastination, you now have different tools to be more productive. To be productive means that you are doing what you said you would do, and usually in a specific time frame.

Observe and check your habits and routines, and then create a productive mindset to get more done in a day. I know you can and will achieve more. So set yourself up to be successful with a prosperous start by following these simple methods.

Printed in Great Britain
by Amazon